Gwen

ewen

IMAGINE A RAINBOW

A Child's Guide for Soothing Pain

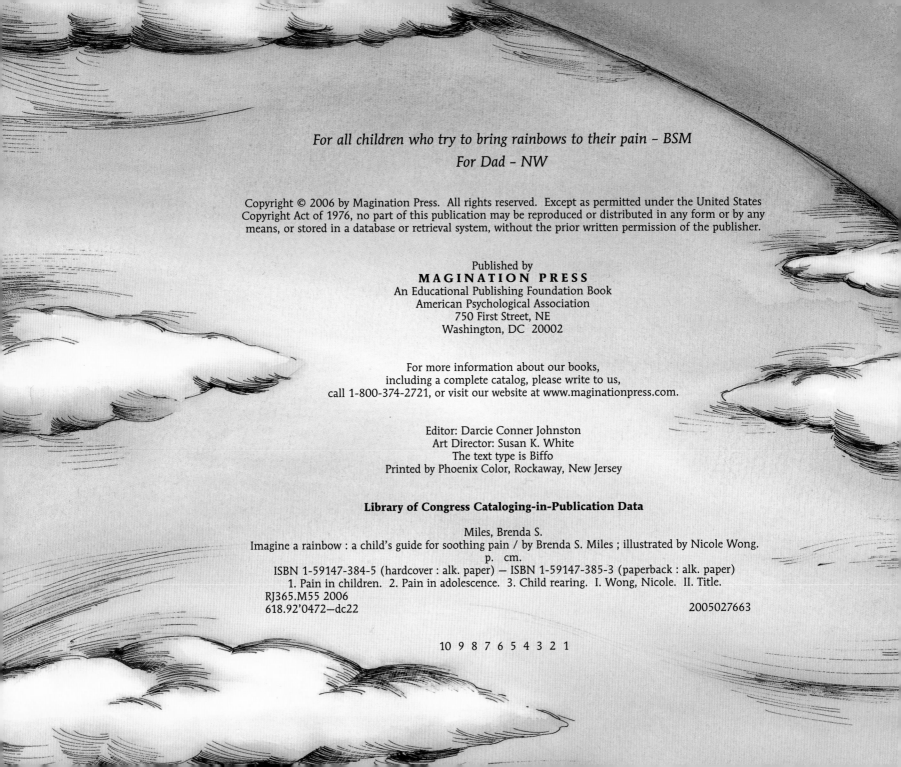

For all children who try to bring rainbows to their pain – BSM

For Dad – NW

Published by

M A G I N A T I O N   P R E S S

An Educational Publishing Foundation Book
American Psychological Association
750 First Street, NE
Washington, DC 20002

For more information about our books,
including a complete catalog, please write to us,
call 1-800-374-2721, or visit our website at www.maginationpress.com.

Editor: Darcie Conner Johnston
Art Director: Susan K. White
The text type is Biffo
Printed by Phoenix Color, Rockaway, New Jersey

Library of Congress Cataloging-in-Publication Data

Miles, Brenda S.
Imagine a rainbow : a child's guide for soothing pain / by Brenda S. Miles ; illustrated by Nicole Wong.
p. cm.
ISBN 1-59147-384-5 (hardcover : alk. paper) — ISBN 1-59147-385-3 (paperback : alk. paper)
1. Pain in children. 2. Pain in adolescence. 3. Child rearing. I. Wong, Nicole. II. Title.
RJ365.M55 2006
618.92'0472—dc22   2005027663

10 9 8 7 6 5 4 3 2 1

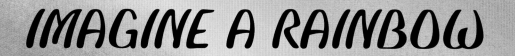

IMAGINE A RAINBOW

A Child's Guide for Soothing Pain

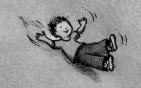

written by Brenda S. Miles, Ph.D.
illustrated by Nicole Wong

MAGINATION PRESS • WASHINGTON, D.C.

You are a child. It doesn't seem fair,
That sometimes your body can hurt everywhere.

There's a way to feel better, something children can do.
The ideas in your mind can help you get through.

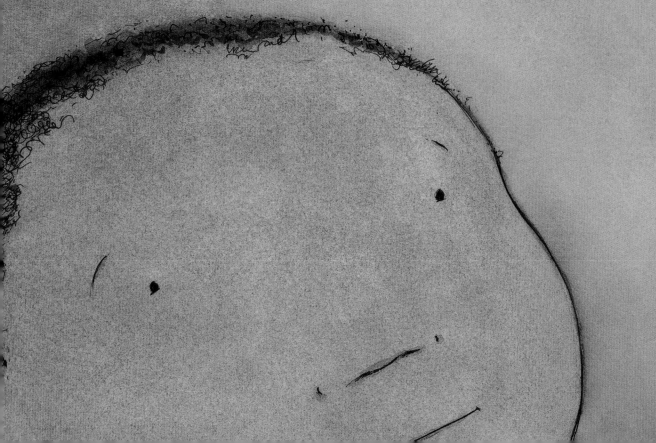

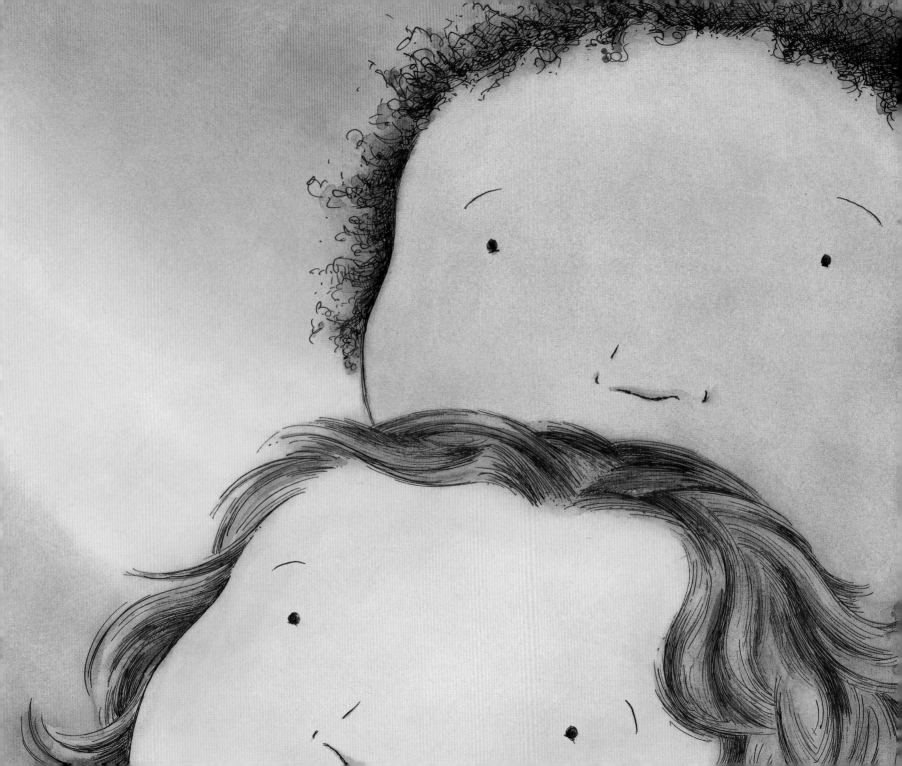

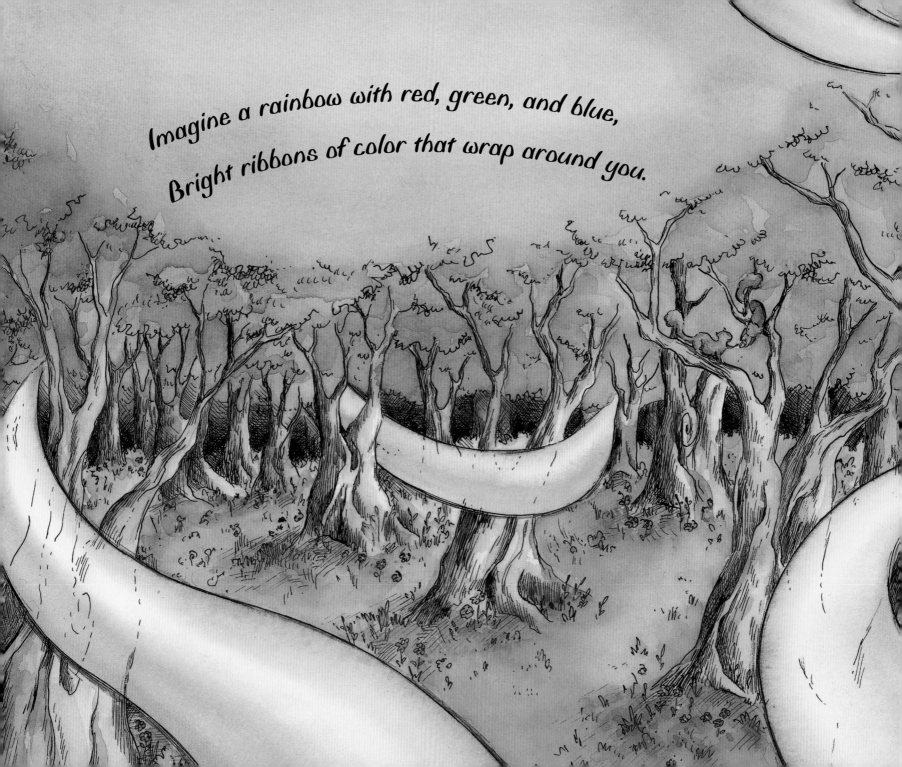

Imagine a rainbow with red, green, and blue,
Bright ribbons of color that wrap around you.

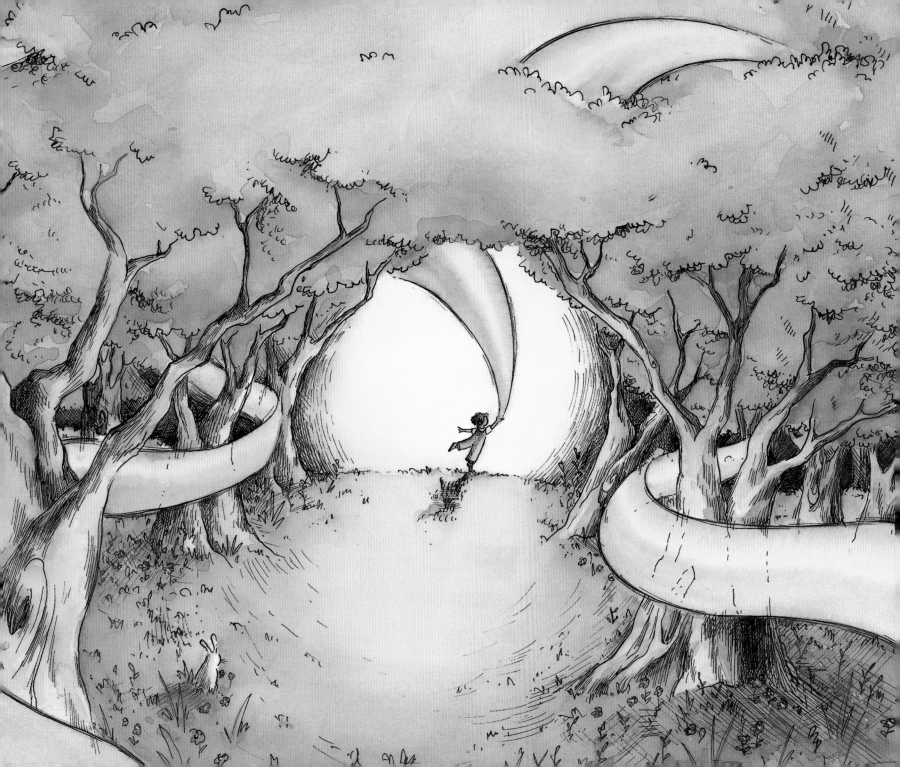

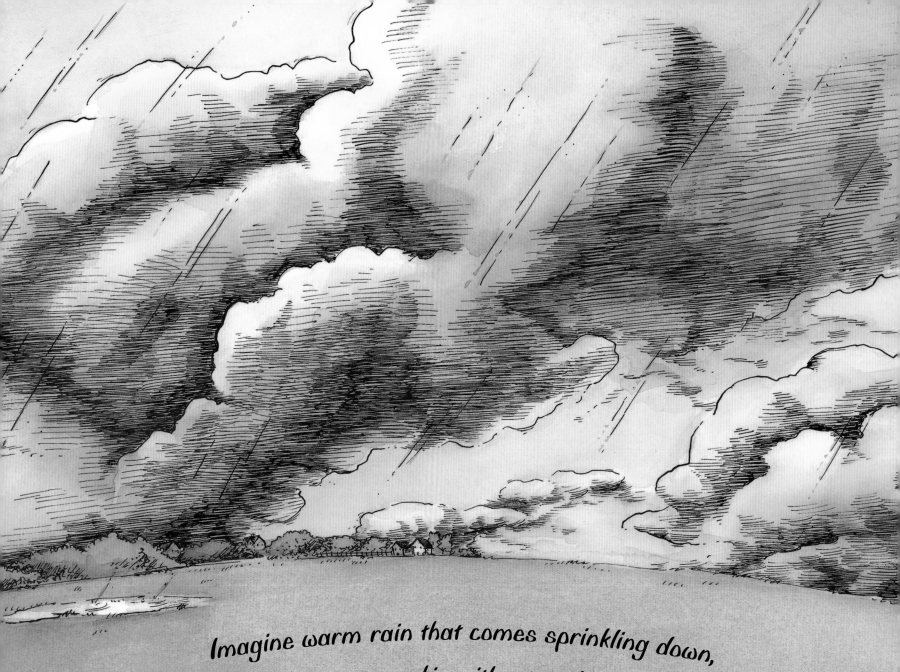

Imagine warm rain that comes sprinkling down,
And kisses your skin without making a sound.

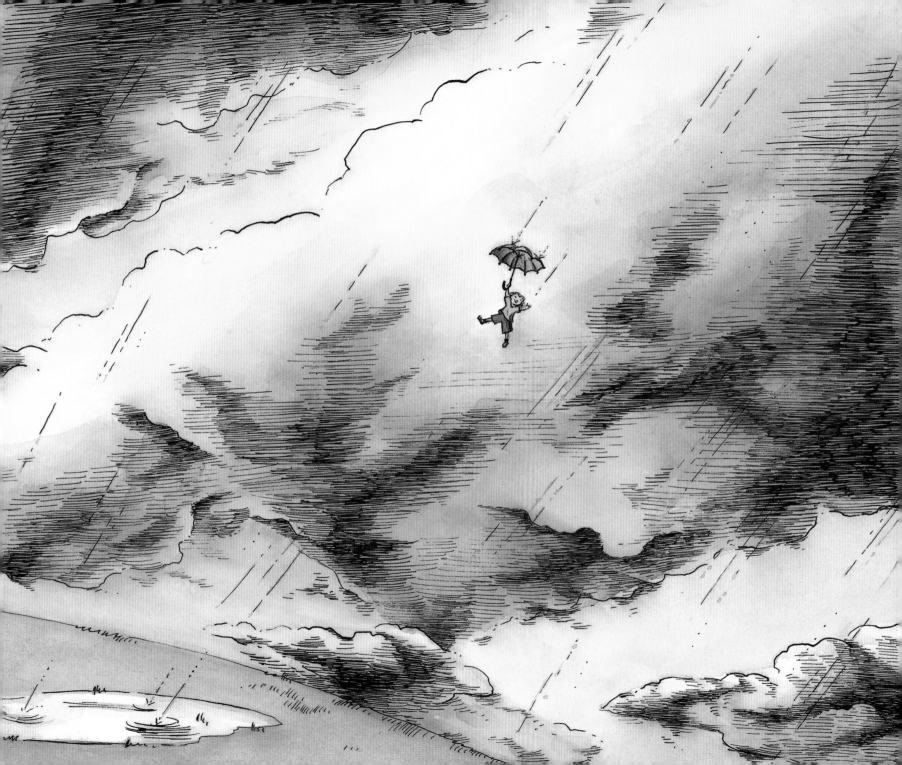

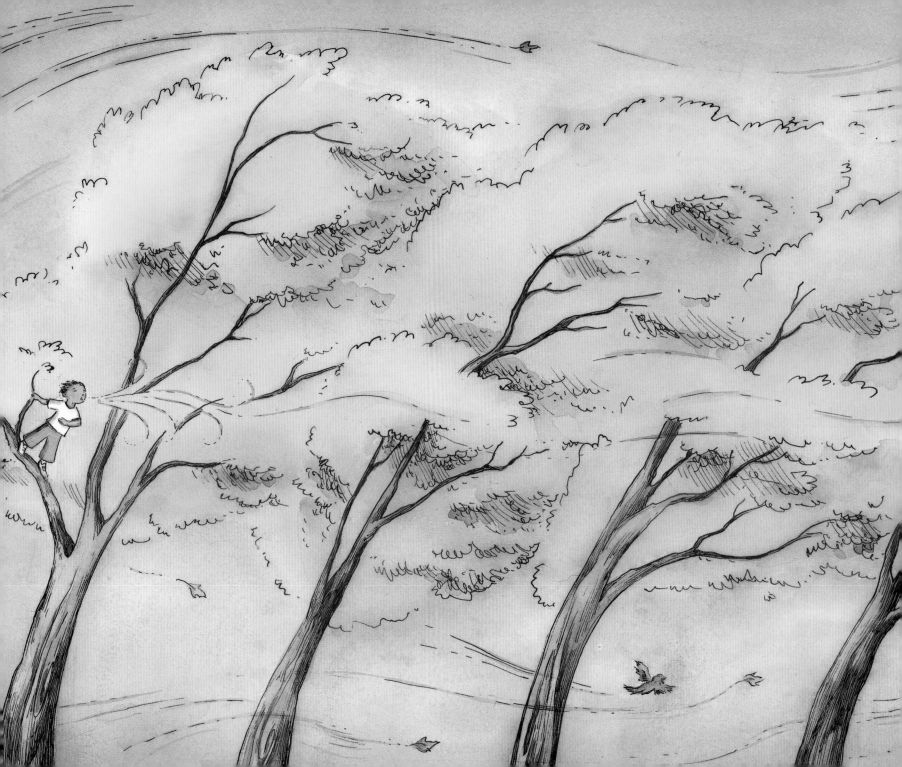

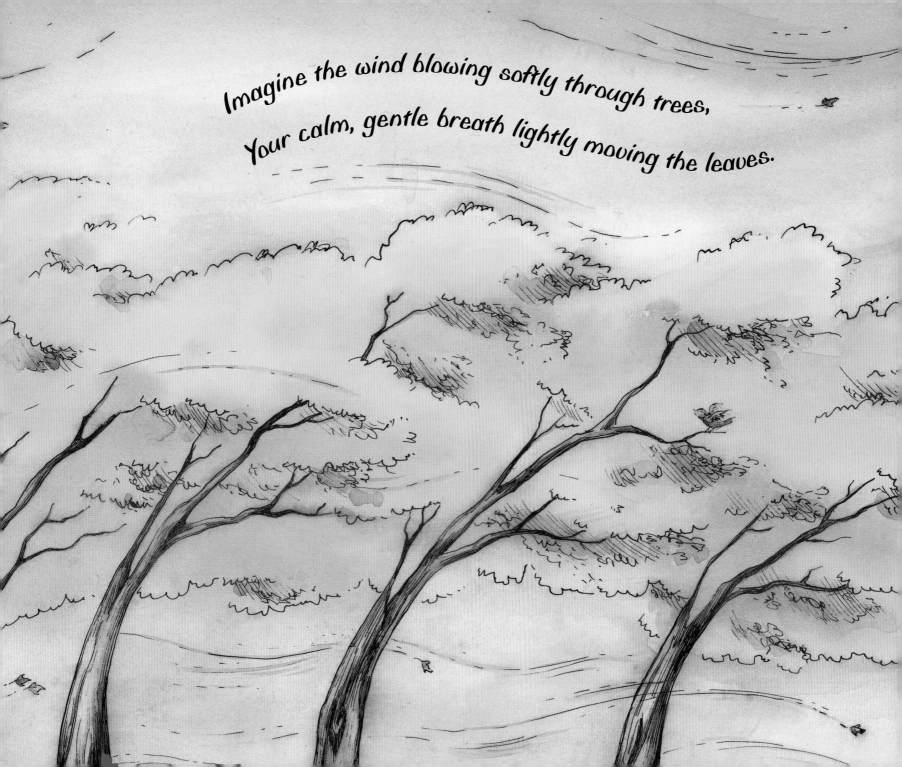

Imagine the wind blowing softly through trees,
Your calm, gentle breath lightly moving the leaves.

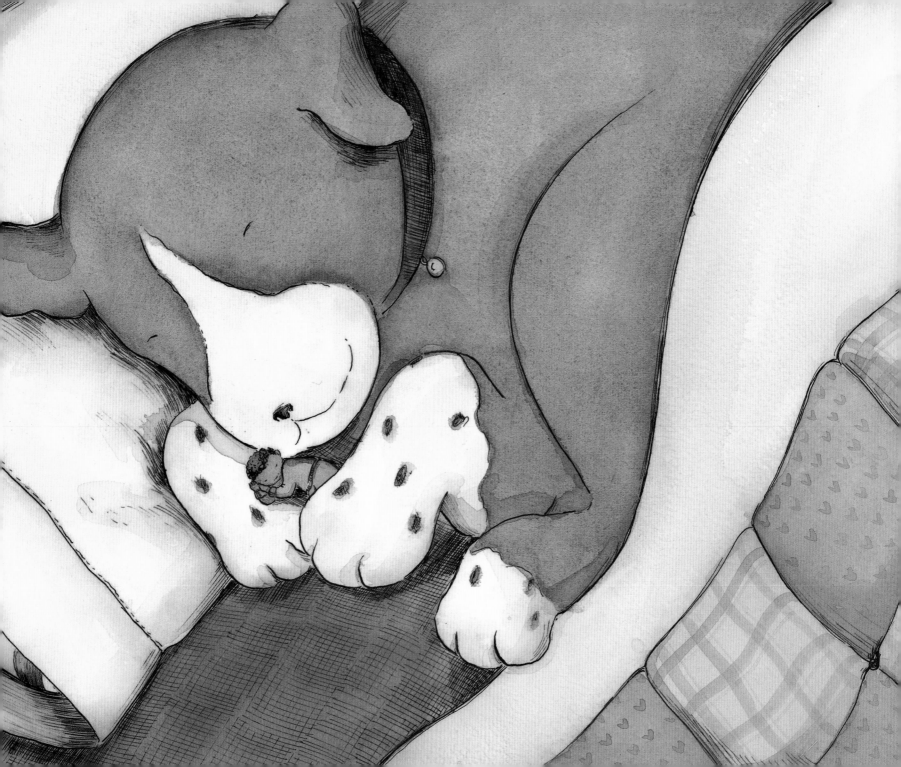

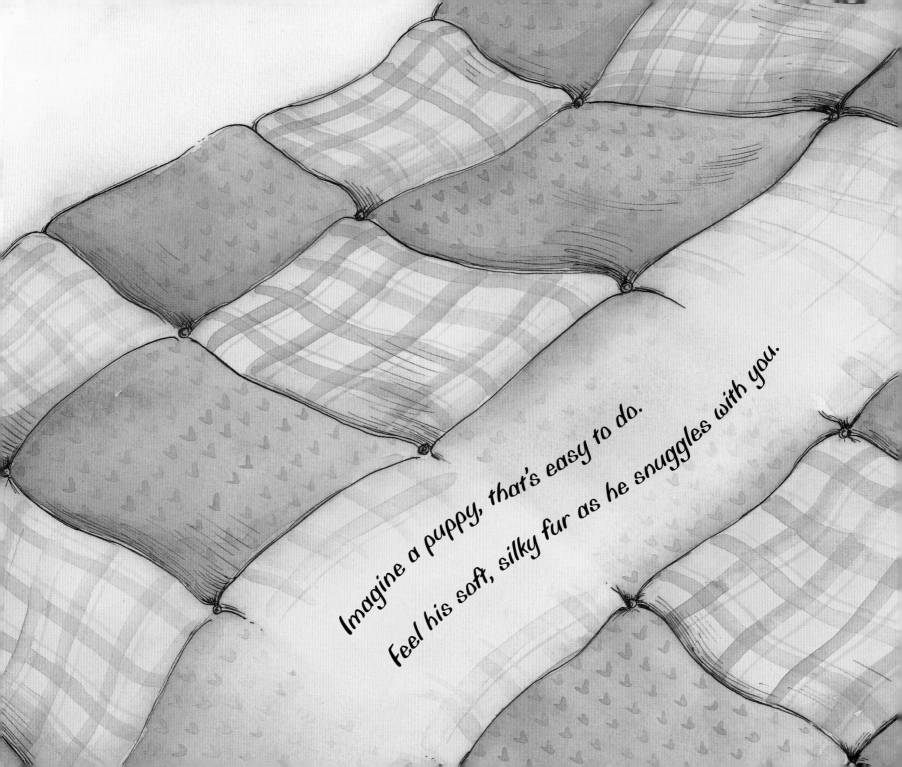

Imagine a puppy, that's easy to do.
Feel his soft, silky fur as he snuggles with you.

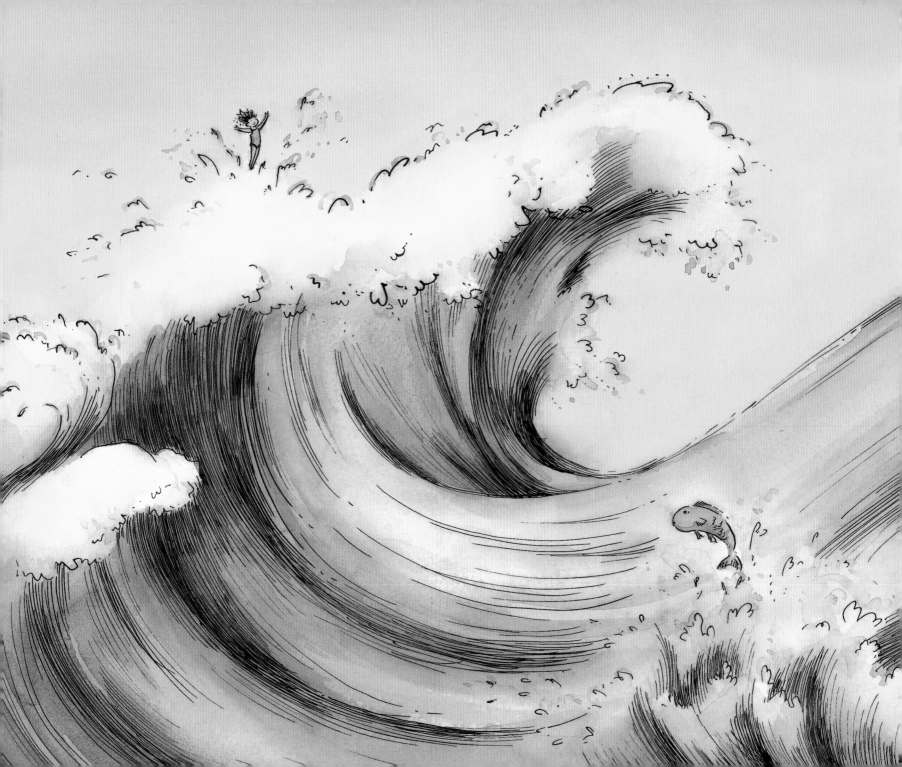

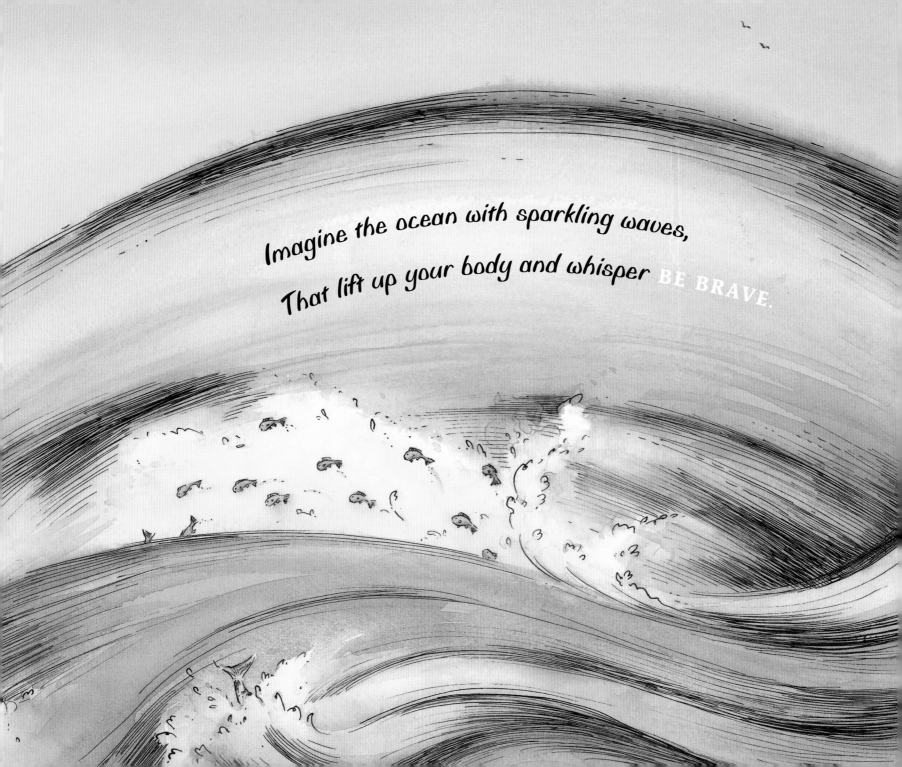

Imagine the ocean with sparkling waves,
That lift up your body and whisper BE BRAVE.

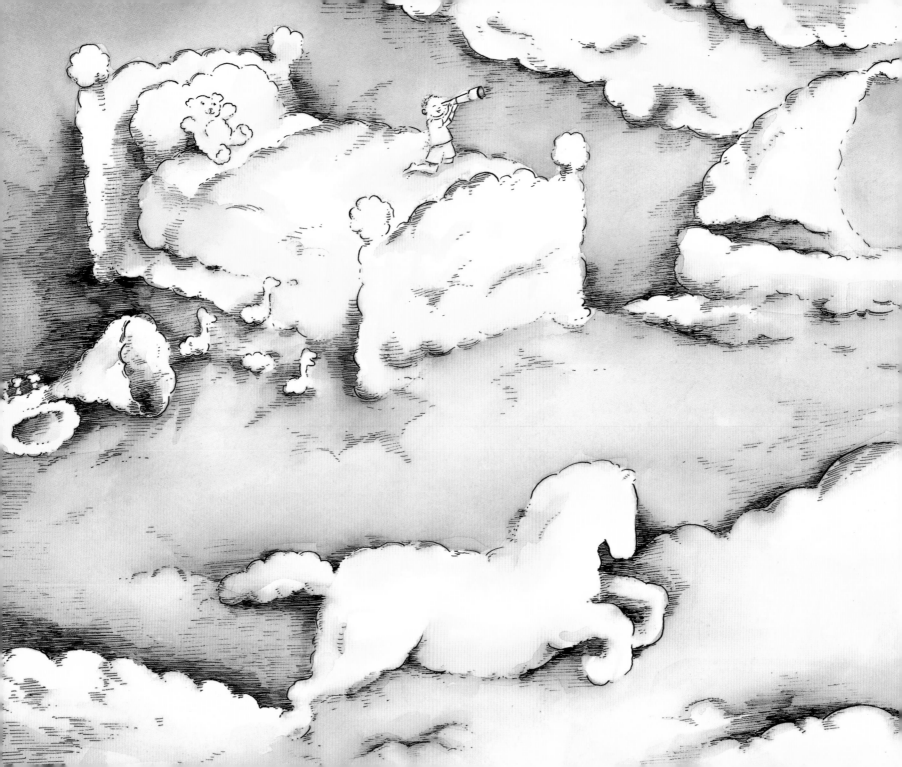

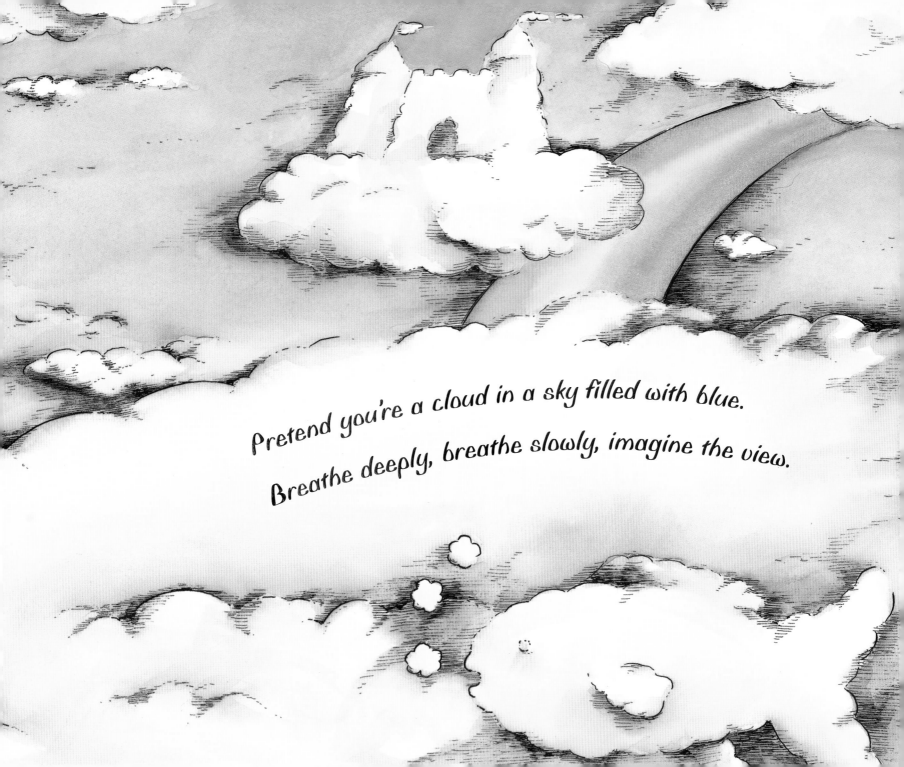

Pretend you're a cloud in a sky filled with blue.

Breathe deeply, breathe slowly, imagine the view.

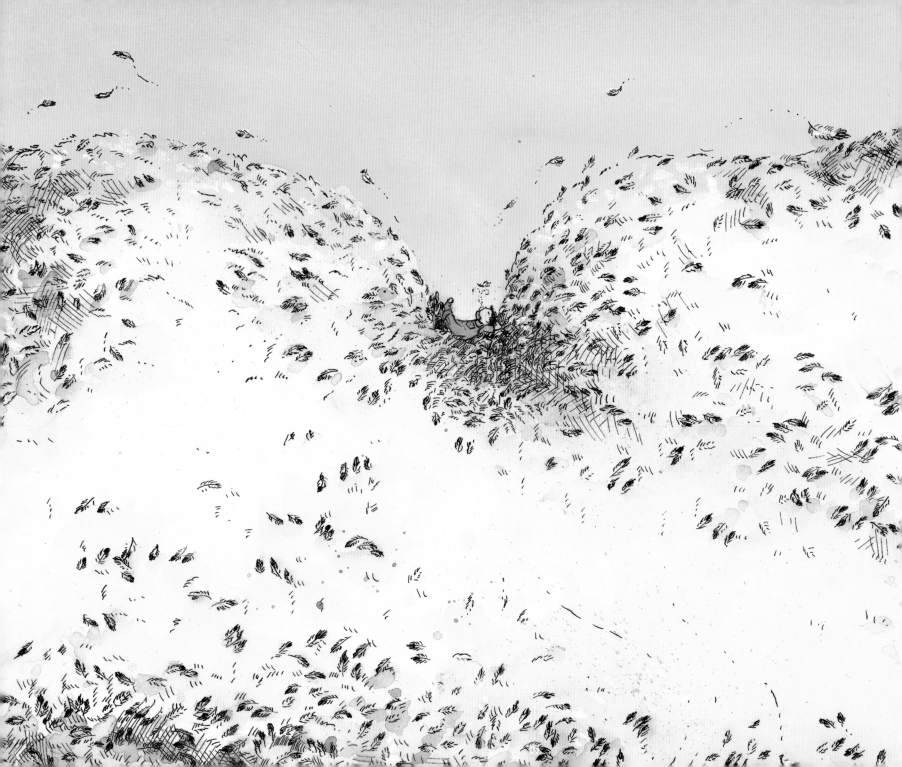

Imagine white feathers stacked twenty feet high,

Such a soft, cozy place for your body to lie.

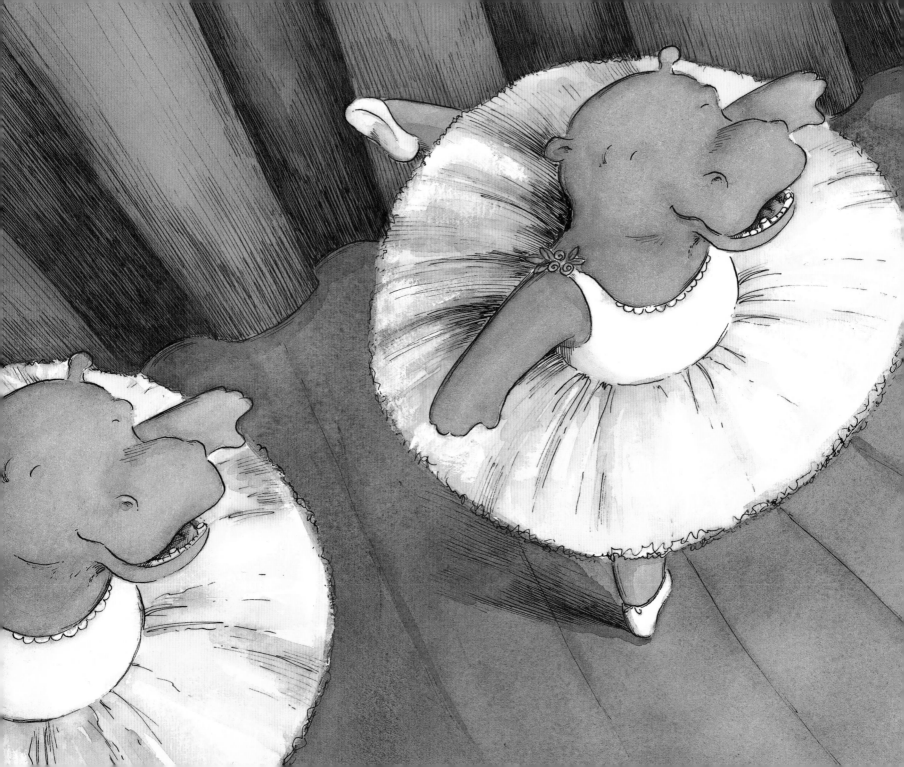

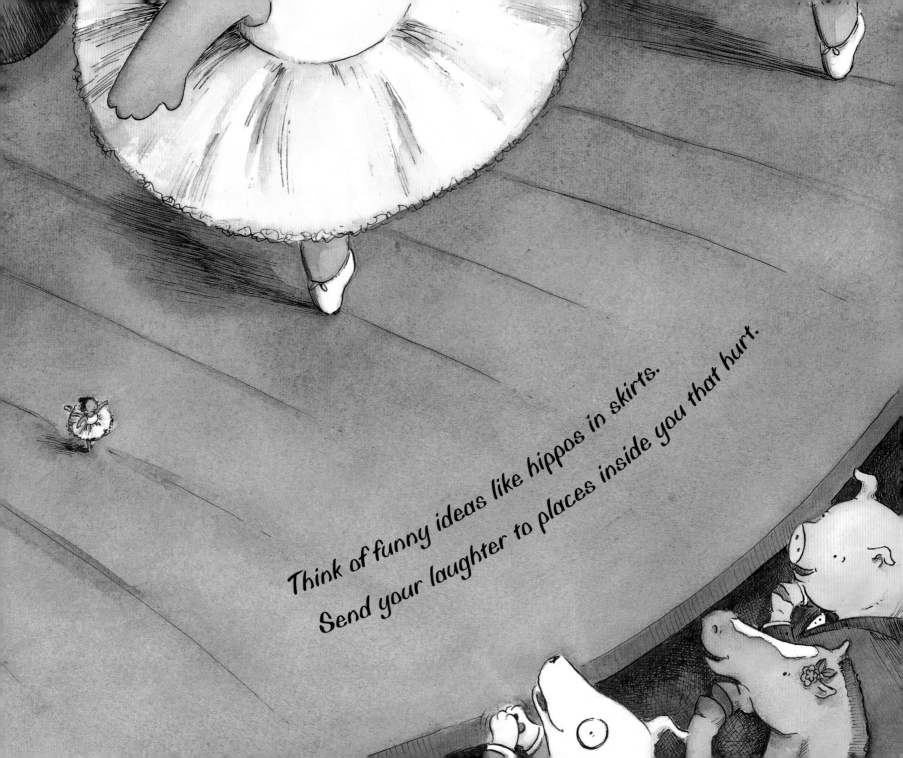

Think of funny ideas like hippos in skirts.
Send your laughter to places inside you that hurt.

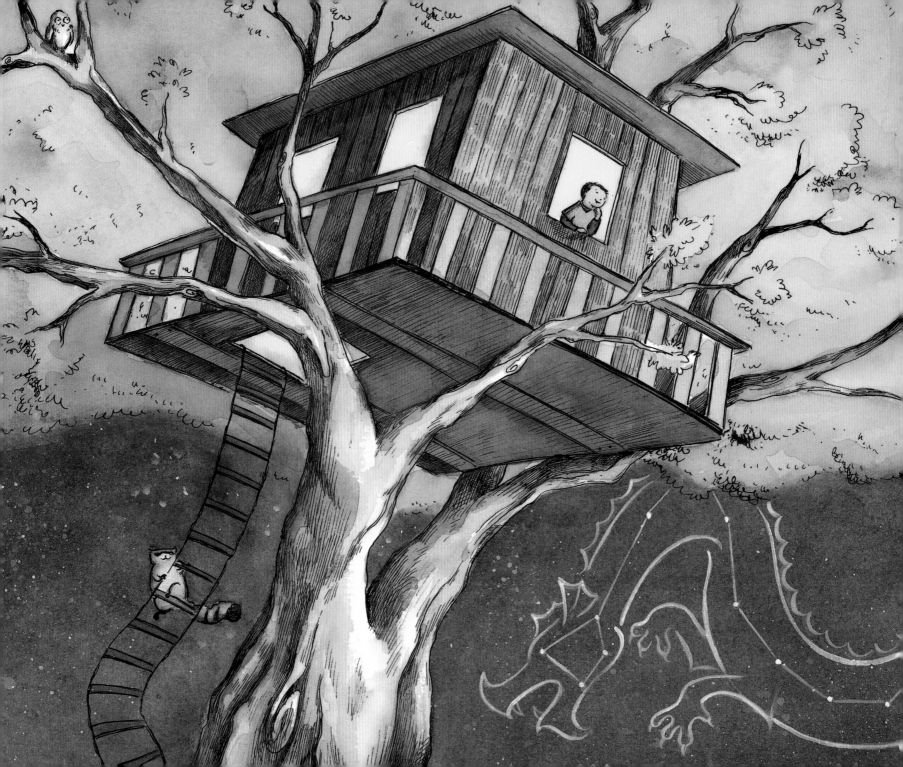

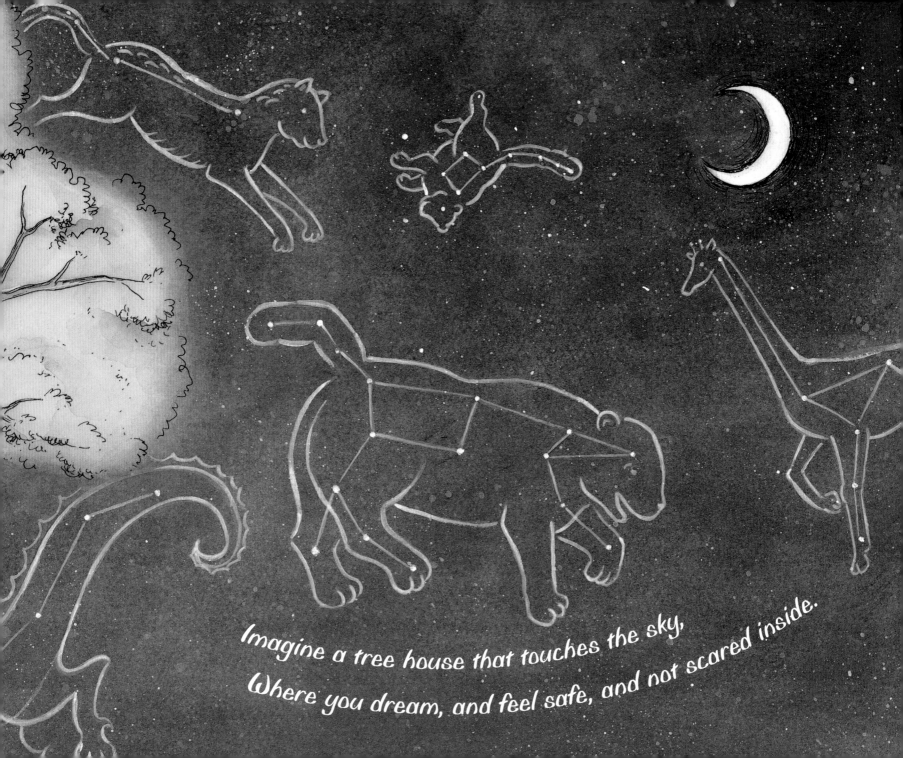

Imagine a tree house that touches the sky,
Where you dream, and feel safe, and not scared inside.

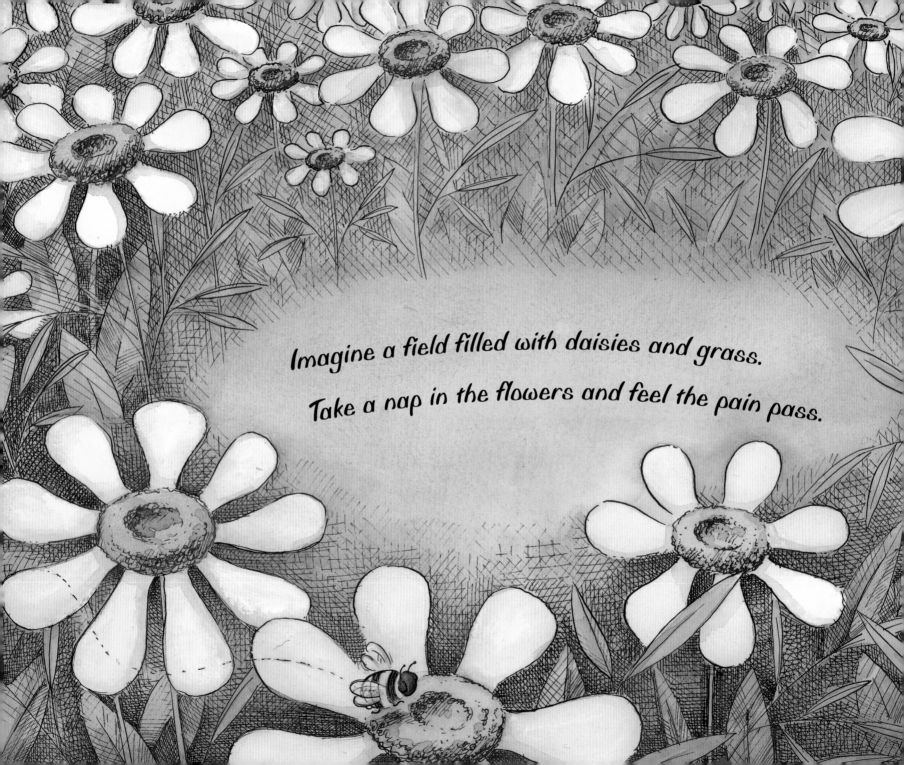

Imagine a field filled with daisies and grass.

Take a nap in the flowers and feel the pain pass.

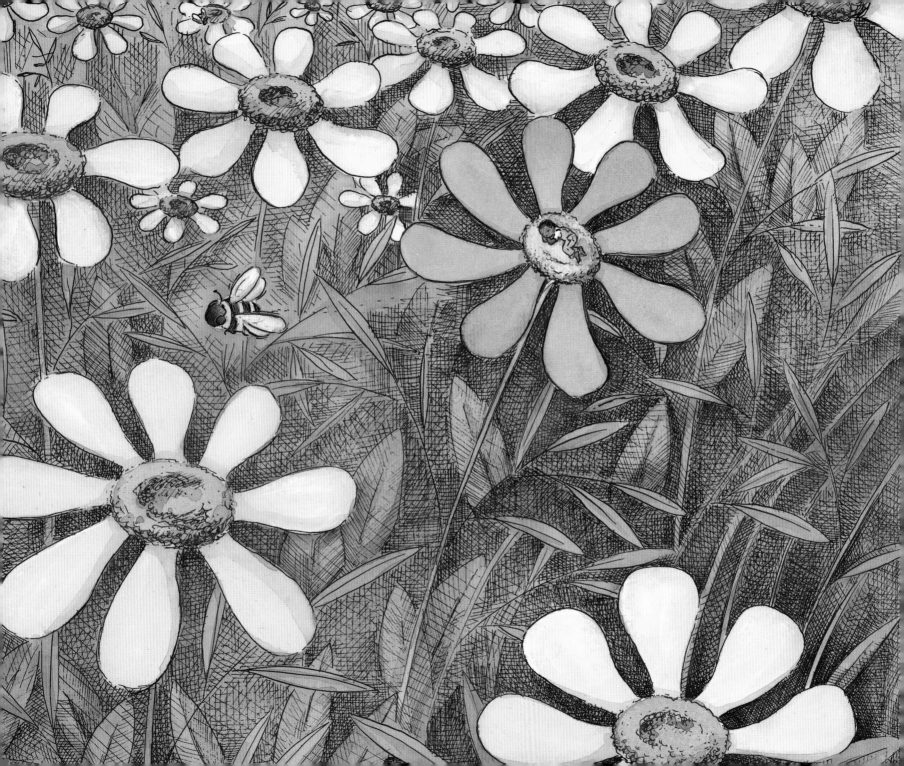

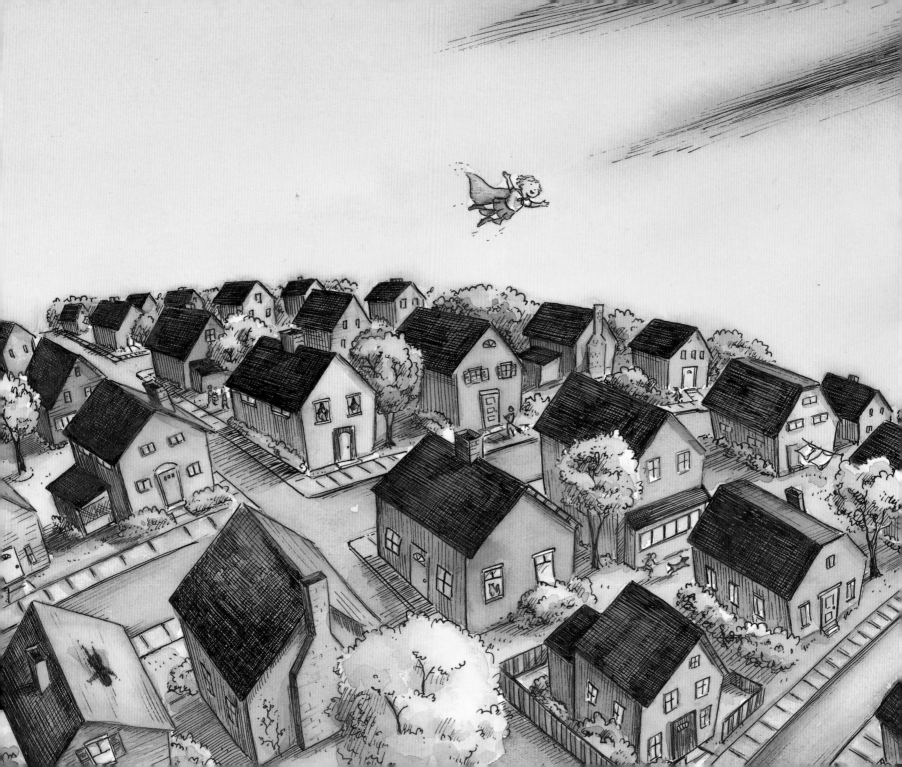

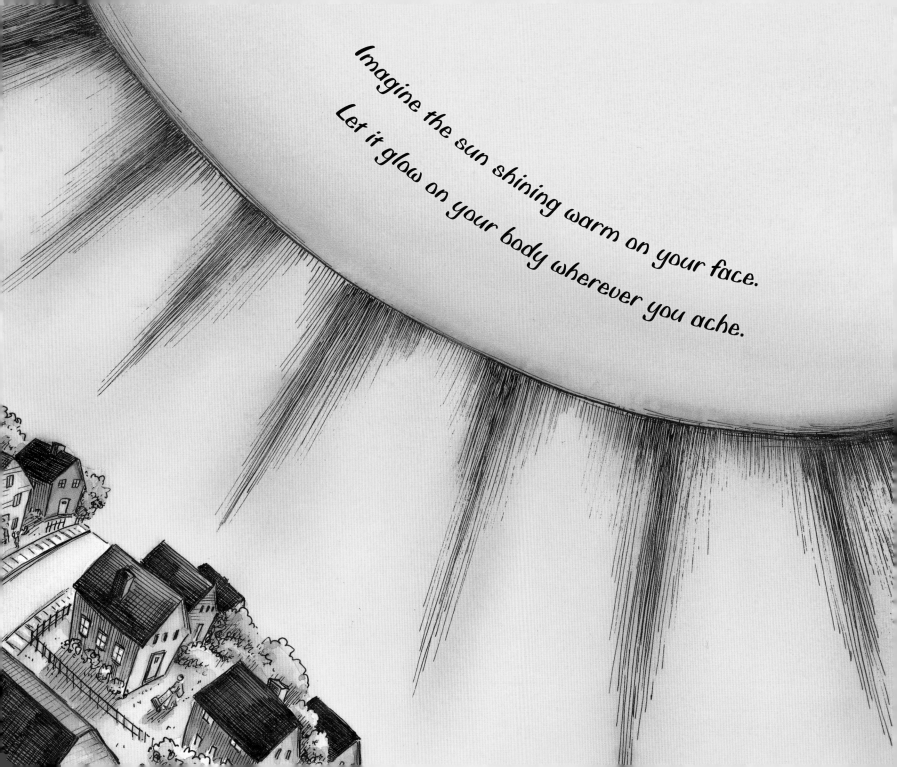

Imagine the sun shining warm on your face.
Let it glow on your body wherever you ache.

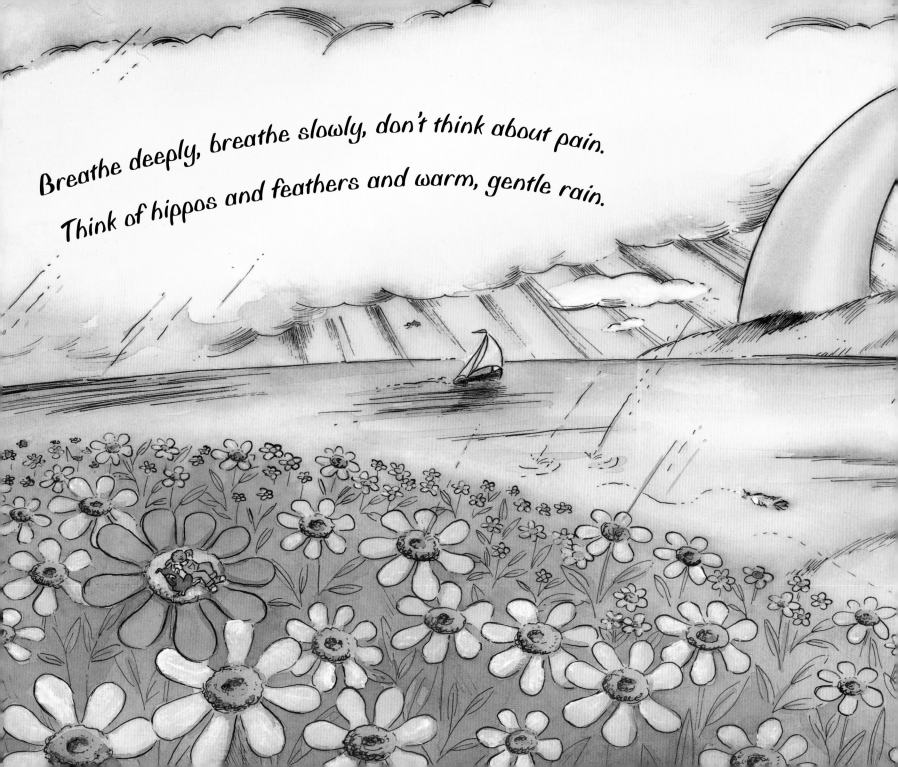

Breathe deeply, breathe slowly, don't think about pain.
Think of hippos and feathers and warm, gentle rain.

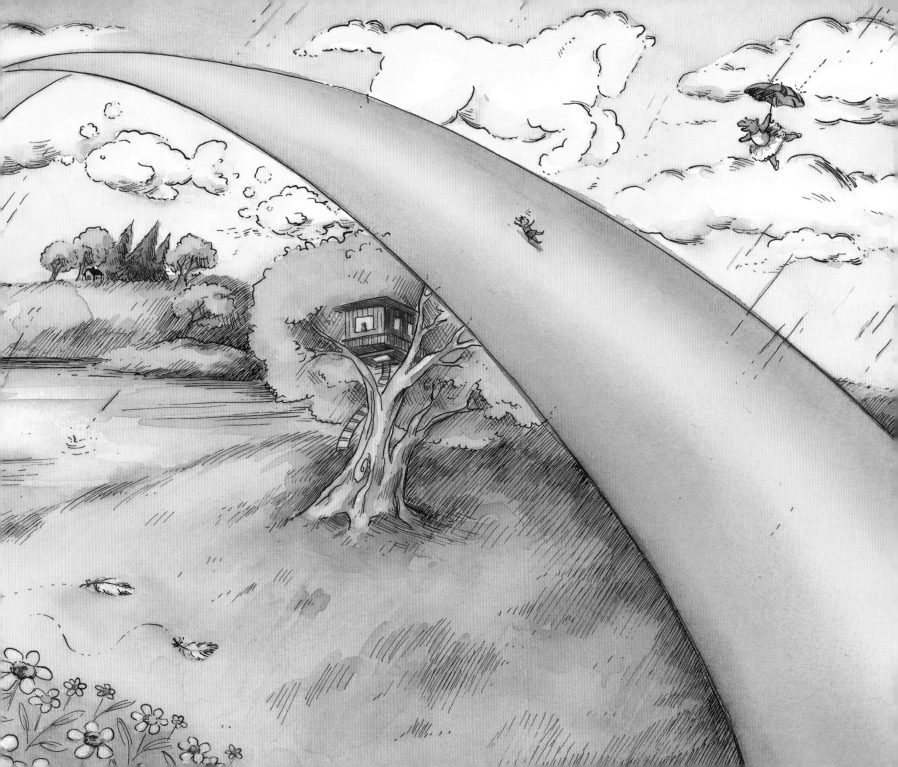

Note to Parents

Childhood is filled with scrapes, bruises, and falls. When a minor injury occurs, children usually shed a few tears, receive a hug and a bandage, and promptly move on. But for some children, pain is a way of life. When a child suffers from something like cancer or sickle cell disease, burns or pediatric arthritis, the management of pain becomes a primary, ongoing concern for both the child and the adults in the child's life.

The purpose of pain is to tell us that a part of the body is hurt, and that it needs attention and protection in order to heal. But pain is more than the biology of nerves sending messages to the brain. A child's experience of pain can also depend on the child's personality, culture, and earlier painful events. It can even depend on the child's expectations of how someone should react when hurt, as parents know from watching a toddler who takes a tumble and then looks to them before deciding whether to cry.

Pain, therefore, has a very real psychological dimension. How a child understands pain, reacts emotionally, and behaves in response to it can heighten or reduce the pain sensation. *Imagine a Rainbow* was written to help children cope with pain by introducing two psychological interventions: **imagery** and **deep breathing.**

IMAGERY

When introducing *Imagine a Rainbow,* tell your child that the book will describe some ways that children can use their imagination when their body is hurting. In age-appropriate terms, explain that thinking about one thing leaves less space in your brain for thinking about other things, such as pain.

You might provide some examples to make this idea more real. For example, you could remind your child of times when he was so interested in an activity that he didn't hear you calling him. Or times when he was so busy he didn't notice he felt hungry, even though it was dinnertime.

As you begin exploring the book together, ask your child to imagine what it would be like to actually be inside the pictures. Explain that the more he can imagine himself this way, the less he will be aware of any pain that might be bothering him. Encourage him to delve into the visual details of each page. If he is particularly fascinated by certain images, focus on these and encourage him to imagine the scene in detail using as many senses as possible. For example, what would a field of daisies *look* like and *smell* like? How would it *feel* to be curled up in a tiny flower, and what would he *hear* as the wind whispers through the petals? Use a gentle and reassuring voice as you discuss the images together.

You and your child may want to return to this book again and again to help reinforce the use of imagination. Continue to talk about the images, and ask him what some of his own relaxing or uplifting "pictures" are. You can help him come up with ideas by volunteering some of your own, and explain how thinking about them helps you feel better. For example, you might say, "When I have a headache, it helps me forget about it when I think about the beach we visit every summer. I can imagine the rushing sound of the waves and the seagulls calling, and I can feel the cool sea breeze on my skin and the warm sand under my bare feet." Help him find and experiment with images he personally finds most comforting and empowering.

DEEP BREATHING

On its own, deep breathing can help a child relax, which can help reduce pain. When combined with imagery, the pair can be even more effective than either technique by itself.

You don't need to wait until your child is in pain to teach deep breathing skills. Explain that when people feel scared, upset, or even in pain, breathing deeply and slowly can help them calm down and feel better. You can also explain that it's a good idea to learn this kind of breathing before it's actually needed. That way, when your child does need it, it's right there, ready for use.

When teaching this skill, start by asking your child to find a comfortable position. She can be sitting up or lying down. Then you might say, "First, blow all of the air out of your lungs.... Now, breathe in s-l-o-w-l-y until your tummy feels full of air.... Now breathe out slowly, until your tummy muscles have pushed all of the air out of your body."

She might imagine her abdomen as a balloon that is first filled with air and then completely deflated. Breathing in and out in this way, using the abdomen rather than the chest, is most effective for relaxing the body. If possible, she should breathe in through the nose and slowly out through the mouth. Her breathing should follow a regular, relaxed rhythm. Breathe with your child to demonstrate the technique and set the right pace, and speak with a soft, gentle voice.

At first she may need the room or space to be quiet as she tries to relax through deep breathing, but with practice she will be able to use this relaxation tool more easily when and where it is needed.

COPING WITH CHRONIC OR RECURRENT PAIN

It is important for children to feel they have some control over their pain. This is especially true when the pain is chronic (such as pain associated with pediatric arthritis, severe burns, or cancer) or recurrent (pain that comes and goes, like the severe pain crises of sickle cell disease). Total pain relief may not be possible in these instances, but children feel less anxious and fearful if they know there is some-thing they can do themselves to lessen their discomfort.

Encourage your child to discuss the pain openly. Some children may hesitate, believing you expect them to be "grown-up." Boys may also be more reluctant than girls to admit that something is hurting. Explain to your child that being brave does not mean denying pain. Instead, it means talking about it and making plans together to feel better. Ask specific questions, such as, "When did the pain start?" "Where does it hurt?" and "What does it feel like?" For younger children, you may need to provide some options for describing the pain, such as "sharp like needles" or "hot and burning."

Imagery and deep breathing can be helpful on their own in instances of mild pain or during procedures that entail brief and minimal discomfort. Chronic or recurrent pain requires more comprehensive pain management that can include medication, as well as psychological and physical techniques developed in consultation with a healthcare team. Although pain medications can be effective, imagery, deep breathing, and other strategies that give your child some control are important additional tools.

COPING WITH MEDICAL PROCEDURES

Fear makes pain worse. In cases of pain related to medical procedures, such as injections and biopsies, a child who has learned what to expect may be especially anxious and in need of pain management strategies. Avoid making promises that a medical procedure won't hurt when in truth it will. False messages can confuse children and, in the long run, increase their fear and anxiety as well as their pain.

Try relating the discomfort of an upcoming medical experience to something familiar or imagined. For example, telling children they may feel tingling for a specific procedure, like the pins and needles they feel in their toes on a cold winter day, may reduce some worry.

Practice imagination and breathing techniques together

with your child before a procedure. You can recite the rhymes in this book together and discuss the images before, during, and after the procedure in order to promote relaxation, reduce anxiety, and enhance your child's feelings of self-control and coping. You may need to work closely with healthcare professionals, such as psychologists, to come up with strategies for relaxation and imagination during complex, painful procedures such as lumbar punctures.

PRACTICING THE SKILLS

Children should be taught that they can use their imagination and deep breathing techniques anywhere and anytime, even without you. Practice will help strengthen these skills. Read this book together and help your child perform these techniques when he or she is not in pain. Practice will help your child use these techniques independently and spontaneously for comfort and relief.

About the Author

BRENDA S. MILES, Ph.D., is a clinical pediatric neuropsychologist who lives in Toronto, Ontario, Canada. She became interested in pain while working with children who have sickle cell disease, a genetically inherited blood disorder that can produce episodes of intense pain. *Imagine a Rainbow* is her first book for children.

About the Illustrator

NICOLE WONG is a graduate of the Rhode Island School of Design. Her illustrations have been featured in several children's books, magazines, and greeting cards. She lives with her husband and their dog and cat in Massachusetts.